WALK & EAT YOURSELF THIN – HOW TO LOSE WEIGHT WHILE STILL EATING SEVERAL MEALS PER DAY (THE WALKING FOR WEIGHT LOSS & EATING PLAN TO BURN BELLY FAT FAST!)

Introduction

If you want to lose weight from your stomach, you are absolutely not alone. This book will help you to achieve your goal and explain to you how you can still eat at the same time, so no more starvation diets.

The obesity epidemic is growing, not only in America but also in many other countries as well. Being overweight is actually a serious issue as it can lead to various health problems, as well as affecting your self-confidence.

So, let's learn how to get rid of that weight. I myself love to eat, as I'm sure you do to. In the following pages you will learn that you can still eat and lose weight at the same time. There really is no need to be hungry whilst dropping pounds, so you won't have to deal with the annoyance of hunger pangs.

Personally I don't think it's worth being hungry the whole time for the sake of being thin. Food is just too enjoyable for that! Hunger is the body's natural way of telling us that we need to eat, so our instincts tell us to get food inside our stomachs as quickly as possible. So it is not a good idea to ignore our natural instincts - we must listen to our bodies and continue to eat regularly.

It is absolutely true that keeping your stomach full by eating regular meals will actually be beneficial in helping you stick to your healthy eating plan; you will end up reaching your goal a lot faster. This also means no more anguish and feeling grumpy because there will be no more hunger.

Big-name diet plans can be expensive, and everything they offer can easily be done on your own. Likewise, diet pills can be dangerous to your health because they contain lots of chemicals and lots of caffeine. The truth is you can get the same effects by being in control of your own weight loss program, and I'm going to give you lots of tips and tricks that will ensure that you succeed. Try to use your want power rather than your will power, and you will be able to achieve your goal!

The Main Reasons for Unwanted Weight Gain

Fast food is one of the main reasons for weight gain, but eating out at fast food restaurants isn't the only problem. It is also how we choose to eat when at home, and this is mainly due to how busy we all are with home and work life these days. Many people go for the easy option of eating pre-packed ready meals that contain unhealthily high amounts of fat and salt.

Our unhealthy eating is reflected in the youth of today, as 15% of all young people below the age of 19 are overweight. And this number is growing. Slow metabolism, although part of the problem, cannot be entirely to blame. There are ways to work around slow metabolism; the main problem is that we eat the wrong foods.

The truth is losing weight is actually much easier than you think, as the most sustainable method is to simply eat less and exercise more. The reason people don't stick to this is because they want super quick results, but with super quick results they may not be long lasting. It's really all about measuring the size of the portions you eat, food choice and exercise. The main key lies in understanding how your metabolism relates to your weight.

Everything You Need to Know About Metabolism

Let's learn how metabolism directly affects your weight. The truth is metabolism doesn't determine your weight alone, but weight is determined on the balance of calories burned versus calories consumed. If you overload on calories you will gain weight. Likewise, you will lose weight if you consume fewer calories. Therefore, metabolism is both the scale that regulates your energy needs and the engine that burns your calories.

Your body converts food into energy by the process that is your metabolism. The energy that your body needs to function is produced by calories combined with oxygen. Your total energy expenditure is the number of calories your body burns each day. Here is what makes up your total body energy expenditure:

Basic - Your basic functions are covered by your basic metabolic rate. The basics are growing and repairing cells, adjusting hormone levels, circulating blood, breathing and fuel for organs. This is the largest portion of energy used as it takes up two thirds to three quarters of your daily calories. This remains quite consistent for the basics needed.

Processing - A further 10% of your daily calories is used by storing, transporting, absorbing and digesting your food. Similarly to your basic needs, your body's requirement to process food stays quite consistent throughout the day.

Physical - The remainder of calories used are taken up doing physical activity such as going for a walk, playing sports or any other movement. These calories burnt can be controlled depending on how intense and frequent these activities are.

Some people might think that unwanted weight gain is the direct result of having a low metabolism, when in fact it is unlikely that they are directly related. A common reason for weight gain is an energy imbalance, where you are consuming more calories than your body burns. So, what you need to do to lose weight in this instance is to eat fewer calories and do more physical activity to burn more calories.

There are many different things that influence how many calories you require, such as the size of your body, your age and sex. You see, a larger body requires more energy and therefore more calories than a smaller body does. Muscle burns more calories and fat, so the more muscle and less fat you have the higher your metabolic rate will be. As your age increases your muscle mass decreases, and more of your weight is accounted for by fat. Also, the older you get the slower your metabolism becomes, so your calorie needs become reduced.

It is true that men have less body fat and more muscle than women do, so this is why men generally have a higher metabolic rate and burn calories faster than women do. Unfortunately, you can't actually change your own metabolism, but you can easily burn more calories by increasing the amount of exercise you do and building lean muscle.

Your energy needs are influenced by your metabolism, however it's the amount of food you consume and the amount of physical activity you partake in that actually determines the amount you weigh. All you need is the motivation to achieve your goal and the dedication to see it through, so developing the right mindset for long-term success is essential.

How To Achieve Long-Term Success

Like many things in life that we aim towards, developing the correct mindset is vital, because there is a frame of mind that must come into play when you are trying to achieve your goal of weight loss. So, we must arm ourselves with the correct information regarding our diet in order to ensure we succeed.

The right mindset will not only give you the motivation, information and commitment levels that are needed, but it will also help you overcome any temptations that try to derail you along the way. Indeed, having the right frame of mind will not only make your weight loss more exciting, easier and a lot more fun, but it will also allow you to dramatically change your lifestyle so you can live the life you want.

Our subconscious controls many of the habits we have and we are mostly unaware of them, and this is the reason why your subconscious could inadvertently destroy our good intentions. Your mindset controls your thoughts, actions and behaviour, so if we employ certain strategies we can control and steer our behaviour to get the outcome we desire. Replacing our old habits by making new associations linked with our desired outcome will help us greatly to lose weight.

You'll find that the more you try to develop the right mindset the easier it will become, and here are some helpful ways to do so:

- Clearly mark down your goals, and be honest with yourself about what weight you want to be.

- When thinking of your goals, be specific. The more specific they are the more important they will feel.

- Give yourself a deadline, because this will add an extra layer of motivation that will really push you to achieving your goal.

- Be realistic. If you aim way too high, achieving your goal may be out of your reach. So make sure you give yourself enough time to realistically get to where you want to be. To make this even easier, you could break down your goal into smaller chunks, so you could tell yourself how many pounds you want to lose over the next month. Then, when you reach this smaller goal you can just rinse and repeat until you reach your larger end goal.

- Make sure you are doing something, however small, on a daily basis. So, focus is the key here. When they are written down in clear view so you can see them every day they will be on your mind and you'll be focused on achieving them.

- Being committed is probably the most important thing, and always remember this. Never forget your reason why you want to do this in the first place, and this will help you stay committed throughout.

We can't overlook the fact that our metabolism slows down as we age, so transforming our food becomes more difficult if we don't change our eating habits and our exercise habits to make up for this. We're going to have to adjust some lifestyle habits in order to maintain our desired weight. You can absolutely achieve success in weight loss by aiming high and pushing yourself with the correct mindset. You will be able to be the person you want to be and live the life you want to live, and you can make that change by starting right this second.

Why You Don't Need To Pay For Diet Companies or Diet Pills

Although many diet companies have their plus points, they are absolutely not necessary in order to lose weight. First of all, they are rather pricey when you consider that you have to pay for the membership along with the food. While some of these diets claim to produce dramatic results, they can also be dangerous to your health. For example, the Atkins diet lets you drop weight drastically because you're consuming very low carbs. However, being able to keep the weight off with this diet becomes very difficult because you won't be able to keep the weight off once you reintroduce carbohydrates. Also, your cholesterol levels will be higher because you are eating foods that are high in fat. By not eating carbohydrates you'll find that your energy levels will be decreased, leaving you feeling tired and unmotivated because carbs are a way for your body to transform food into energy. It will also be much harder to get a decent pump during a workout, since your muscles will be much softer. A diet plan that balances out everything you need to operate your body at an optimal level is a diet plan worth doing.

Similarly, diet pills have risks associated with taking them. Because these pills do not need to be tested by the Food and Drug Administration, they can be loaded with health risks. Even if a pill is found to be hazardous to your health, the Food and Drug Administration will remove it from future sale, but this doesn't stop it from being available in the first place.

How These Pills Work

Many of these pills suppress your appetite, some claim to increase your body's ability to burn fat and reduce hunger, while others claim to help you lose weight by removing the body's fluids. They can also be addictive, as well as having the following undesired effects: sex drive disturbances, excessive sweating, blurred vision, dizziness, headaches, fever, high blood pressure, anxiety and many more.

Nothing makes you lose weight more effectively like a balanced diet and exercise. Doing it the natural way will help you grow emotionally and improve your lifestyle.

Why Balance Is Important

It's good to drink a lot of water. A lot of people don't drink as much as they need. You should really drink eight glasses of water a day, or possibly more. You see, water is a natural appetite suppressant. So if you drink a full glass of water before you consume a meal, your stomach won't need as much food to feel full. And drinking water will not make you gain weight, instead it will hydrate your body. When we don't drink enough water, and then suddenly drink a lot we start to feel bloated. So it's much better to drink it gradually throughout the day so that it's released naturally. Then you can get the added bonuses of hydration and a feeling of fullness.

The basic food groups that make up a balanced meal is what you should always aim for. As carbohydrates are the main source of energy while proteins burn fat, each meal should include a protein and a carbohydrate. Skipping meals is extremely detrimental in regards to weight loss because your metabolism needs regular meals to stay consistent. Your body thinks that it's starving if you have an erratic eating schedule, so when you do eat it stores it as fat so it can be used for energy.

Living a sedentary lifestyle and losing weight isn't possible. People who exercise lose weight more quickly than those that don't, they also live longer and generally feel better about themselves. This doesn't have to be a vigorous gym routine, but can instead be something as simple as walking for weight loss.

The simple formula to help you calculate weight loss is: intake fewer calories than what you burn on a daily basis. So, consuming 2000 calories and burning 2500 calories in one day is ideal. Cutting down loads on the amount of calories you intake so that you won't need to burn as many is not a good way to lose weight because you will be starving yourself. You'll feel weak and hungry, and you won't be eating yourself thin.

Your body needs energy, and it needs food and calories to get this energy. Thus, eating enough so you're not starving and being able to burn off what you've eaten and a bit more afterwards is key. However, if the amount of calories you burn is the same as the amount of calories that you intake, you will remain the same.

So, the simple way to lose weight and eat at the same time is to make the correct choices when it comes to food. You need to select foods that have a low calorie count but can also satisfy your hunger. Research has shown that fat contains 9 calories per gram compared to protein and carbohydrates which contain 4 calories per gram, so the more fat contained in a food the more calories. The weight of the food you eat may very well play a more significant part in satisfying hunger than fat or calories. Thus, eating high calorie or high-fat foods to feel full may not be needed but instead your stomach needs to feel weighted by a certain amount of food.

People have a tendency to eat the same weight of food on a daily basis, no matter of the amount of fat or calories that the meal contains. Your stomach has a weight that needs to be filled for you to feel full when eating. This is why consuming soup or having a glass of water before a meal reduces your appetite, and it is also why people can consume a low-fat diet and still gain weight if most of their foods are carbs and starch.

How To Eat Yourself Thin

Eating food based on the weight to calorie ratio is key to eating for weight loss. So avoid food that is full of calories and light in weight, and instead choose food that has a low calorie count but weighs a lot. The best ones to go for are vegetables and fruits, as they are heavy due to their water and fibre content plus they are low in calories.

Snack foods, although not weighing much contain a lot of calories. So they are to be avoided because you can consume a lot of them without feeling full and therefore take in a too many calories. Indeed, lightweight food with a high calorie count is arguably the worst food to eat if you are trying to lose weight, because you are not full and you have already consumed more than enough calories. A lot of people when dieting avoid eating regular size meals because they think the larger the meal the more weight they will gain, but they don't see that lightweight foods can be detrimental if high in calories.

In order to eat and lose weight at the same time, we must cut down on our carbohydrates slightly but not entirely. We need some carbs in our system so we can have the energy to partake in exercise - without any carbs in our system this would be much more difficult, and the calories would not get burnt off.

A good balance is to make sure that at least half of your calories come from fruit, vegetables, whole grains and natural starches. Whilst the remainder of your diet should be lean protein like fish and chicken. So, balance your carbs with your protein and avoid eating carbs late at night. If you are feeling lacking of energy on a certain day, you can increase your carb intake briefly to get your energy levels up again.

As far as protein is concerned, a good rule is you should consume 1 gram of protein for every pound of body weight per meal. Although that sounds very high, the protein being referred to is lean protein so there will be hardly any fat intake. It will also accelerate regular weight loss because protein speeds up your metabolism.

When considering portion sizes, it is a good idea to never eat a serving that is larger than your clenched fist. This way you won't be overdoing it and will still feel full. If you start to crave food that you love - for example biscuits, then that's fine as long as you don't overdo it. Instead of eating several, just have one. You don't have to cut out your favourite foods as long as you keep them in moderation.

To combat hunger, you should eat more meals with smaller portions instead of fewer meals with larger portions, because when you are overly hungry you tend to overeat. As far as the smaller portion sizes are concerned, women should eat five meals per day, and men should eat six. Be sure that these meals are at least two hours apart so you'll never crave food. You will soon discover the benefits, such as:

- Better absorption of the nutrients in your food.

- Better utilisation of the nutrients in your food.

- Greater muscle growth.

- Steadier blood sugar and insulin levels.

- Reduced hunger cravings.

- Less storage of body fat.

- Higher energy levels.

- Faster metabolic rate.

Foods You Should Avoid For Weight Loss

Here is a rundown of the foods that you should absolutely avoid for weight loss. These are the worst foods, and some great alternatives.

Pre-packed foods - Basically, anything in a cardboard packet you should stay away from especially if the ingredients are not pronounceable. This is because they contain a lot of chemicals which are going to be detrimental to your diet and health. Although white rice is filling, it contains a lot of starch that can slow down your weight loss, so eat brown rice instead. Another food that contains a lot of starch is pasta mixes, so instead consume whole grain pasta - it's just as tasty and much healthier.

Drinks - You should avoid sodas and anything with caffeine in it. This is because caffeine has an insulin-stimulating weight loss inhibiting effect, so stick to decaffeinated soft drinks, coffees and teas. Likewise, stay away from any beverage that contains aspartame, refined sugar or high fructose corn syrup. Because you will be drinking water as part of your weight loss plan, a slice of lemon or lime in it can add a lot of flavour.

It's okay to have one alcoholic drink with dinner, as long as you don't drink more than this because alcohol is detrimental in regards to weight loss. Even alcoholic beverages that say they have fewer calories will still make you gain weight, so moderation is essential.

Bread - White bread is also high in starch so should be steered clear of. You will still find the carbohydrates you need in whole grain bread and they are less processed. Instead of just wheat flour, make sure the bread you choose is made with whole-wheat flour, for this will make a lot of difference.

Cans and jars - Canned food and jarred food needs to be free from a lot of chemicals. Many soup mixes are very fatty, as is chicken broth, so avoid them. Luckily there are a lot of low-fat or light choices available, so go for these. There is a tremendous amount of salt and sugar in readymade tomato-based sauces, so the best option is to make your own. Don't consume canned vegetables or canned fruit, because it's already been cooked therefore has lost almost all of its good nutrients. They also have a lot of processed sugars so always stick to fresh vegetables and fresh fruit. As far as oil goes, go for extra virgin olive oil instead of any corn-based or vegetable oils.

Protein - Lean meats are the only choice because of their low-fat. Red meat isn't as good for you as white meat, but if you do eat it pick out a lean cut with the portion size no larger than your clenched fist. When it comes to fish, fresh fish is always the way to go instead of canned, and go for the lower fat types such as cod, tuna and salmon. Grilling your fish is the best way to get rid of any remaining fat, and avoid the battered or breaded variety. There is much less fat in white meats such as chicken and turkey, rather than red meat.

Milk, Cheese and Eggs - Try not to drink too much milk because it contains some facts that can lead to weight gain. But skimmed milk is the way to go over any other kind. Alas, cheese contains fat so it's not going to help your diet, but low-fat or fat-free is okay in moderation. It's fine to eat eggs, as they are high in protein but try to only use the whites and not consume the yolks. Yoghurt is desirable over cream, although fat-free sour cream is okay if used sparingly.

Fruit and veg - Luckily pretty much all fresh vegetables will do you good, and therefore you can eat as much as you want and you'll still lose weight. Steamed is the best way to cook them, followed by oven baking or grilling. As far as fruit is concerned, be wary of fruits that contain a lot of natural sugars. Peaches and oranges are two examples of these. Even though the sugar is natural, try not to consume too much because it will still be converted to fat.

When embarking on a new diet a great psychological trick is to throw out all foods that could be tempting and potentially sabotaging to your good intentions. So get rid of the processed sugar, frozen ready meals and chips.

Your New Healthy Shopping List

Making a list before you go shopping for your new diet is an excellent technique in making sure you don't get tempted and buy food that is going to be detrimental to your weight loss. Make sure you stick to your list and plan wisely and you won't slip up.

Once you decide what your new healthy meals are going to be, picking out the ingredients needed to prepare them will be easy. Just remember to include portion sizes when planning, as this is key to consistent weight loss. Because you'll be eating several smaller meals in a day, be sure to include all the meals that you'll need.

It's a great idea to eat before you go grocery shopping. Unwanted purchases tend to happen if you're hungry when food shopping, so you won't fall into this trap if you eat before you go.

Read the labels before you buy the products, so you don't get food that will be bad for your diet. Always peruse the salt, sugar and fat content, so that you're sure you're buying food that is weight friendly. Steer clear of the pre-packed meals in the frozen section, because even though they are convenient they contain many fats and additional unneeded calories.

Cooking your own meals is the way to go, and preparing from scratch is the best option. This way you will have total control over what exactly goes into your food, the amount of sugar or salt, and it'll be tastier too.

When shopping, just remember to always stay away from food that contains empty calories such as sweets, biscuits and french fries. They will give you no nutritional value, so avoid them at all costs. Follow this plan plus exercise, and you will find that you don't have to starve yourself at all in order to lose weight.

How to Optimise Losing Belly Fat by Walking

Couple the exercise of walking with the eating for weight loss techniques explained in the earlier parts of this book and you'll absolutely succeed in reaching your goal. You can dramatically change the shape of your body just by walking 10,000 steps, and this section will guide you on your way to becoming a fitter, healthier you. This simple exercise is easy on the joints and guaranteed to shed pounds and burn belly fat. You just need to stay focused on your goal and take a walk at least twice a week.

The Process of Walking to Burn Fat

Walking is a fail-proof way to alter your exercise habits. There's no gym membership, extra costs or special skills required – all you need is the open road.

Once you get into the habit of walking, you'll find that you'll still be able to eat your favourite foods. Burning off the fat will become second nature - all you need to do is put on your walking shoes and burn the fat off. It's all about routinely following an exercise program and reaping the long-term rewards.

Although 10,000 steps might at first sound like a long distance, it's actually not that far at all. It's basically just a long stroll. By walking at a steady pace you can complete this distance in about one and a half hours. It's just under five miles in distance. The speed it takes you to complete your walk can be increased dramatically if you power walk. Power walking will change your normal walks into strength training and cardio. If you engage in power walking, it will become possible to complete your 10,000 steps in one hour.

The Clever Way to Drop Pounds

Anyone can achieve their weight loss goals by walking, you just have to stick to it. It actually makes a lot more sense to walk for weight loss rather than put yourself on a strict diet because you won't have to deal with the constant food cravings. The changes you will make by walking will improve your self confidence and help you lead a happier healthier life. Rather than go through the hunger and of not eating it is much easier and more pleasurable to take a walk. When you walk for weight loss you will naturally start to develop healthier eating habits, because you are regularly exercising and you will find that you will naturally want to eat healthier too. A lot of the pressure of weight loss will be eliminated.

The True Reason Why Walking Burns Fat

When you start moving your body, you will straight away start burning fat. Your metabolism will be greatly increased due to your muscles being put into gear. In fact, studies have shown that active people even burn calories when they sleep – so ultimately you will have to do a lot less work in the long run to achieve the body shape you desire. The truth is: you can burn 150 calories in just half an hour of walking. Now, if you start power walking, this can be increased to over 400 calories in one hour. That's a figure that I think we can all be excited about. Plus, fat will continue to be burnt off even after you've finished your walk.

The Easy Way to Walk Further

Walking 10,000 steps isn't easy for everyone, straight away. Many people have to build up to it, and this is totally fine and absolutely normal. The easiest and quickest way to motivate yourself and go the distance is to use a pedometer. This convenient device straps to your leg and counts how many steps you've taken. After each walk, take a look at the amount of steps you've taken and make a serious effort to increase this by 500 steps the next time you do it. Keep this up, and you'll discover that you can walk the full 10,000 with minimal effort within a couple of weeks. This step counting will add a sense of urgency to your new exercise regime, and will also give you a great sense of satisfaction when you hit your targets. Also, your height will determine how many steps you can take in a five mile walk – so using a pedometer will give you a far more accurate number of steps, rather than just walking the miles.

Your Body Mechanics and How This Simple Exercise Sheds Pounds

In order to burn belly fat, your abdominal muscles need to be engaged. This is why walking burns belly fat – because when you do this low-impact exercise you are actually engaging your whole body including your abs. Your posture and a steady speed both help the process, because the easy effort of maintaining a straight posture will draw your core in, thus building toned muscle on your stomach. While doing this, your body will burn up fat to use as energy, and this includes your obliques because the opposite limb movements we all naturally do when walking helps to get rid of the unwanted fat at the sides of our body. Performing crunches will no longer be necessary as walking can be used to replace these tiring exercises, and can actually be far more effective, with no risk of hurting your lower back. An added bonus of this is protecting your spine. When your abdominals become stronger from walking, the opposite side of your core – the spine – will be under far less stress when lifting heavy things.

Quick Fat Burning Facts

- During your walks, longer strides will dramatically increase your body's fat burning capabilities.
- Increasing the speed of your walking will increase the toning of your abdominals.
- You are sure to shed more pounds walking fast than the same person would walking at a slower speed.
- Power walking forces you to tighten your abs and they remain tightened until you have finished.
- This increases your body's natural capabilities of burning fat because you are actually changing your body's chemical balance that in turn results in you being conditioned to burn fat.

- The whole process becomes easier and easier, resulting in less effort to maintain a toned midsection.

- After your walk while you are recovering, the process of after-burn with continue to burn those calories.

Good for the Mind As Well As the Body

Walking for exercise is also a great way to decrease our daily stresses and help to clear our mind. It also enhances our spirit and enthusiasm for life. An unusual fact is that people that suffer from stress actually retain more fat than people that have a more easy-going disposition. The reason for this is because of their increased level of cortisol. So, by exercising you will reduce your stress levels and also decrease your cortisol. With being active and healthy it's a case of the better it gets, the better it gets. Meaning you'll be able to keep the weight off whilst simultaneously maintaining a well-balanced mood.

Tips on Walking Fast

Before you embark on power walking, it's a good idea to make sure you have the correct footwear. This is important because when walking for exercise your feet need to have a good range of motion particularly in the mid part of the foot. Tracksuit bottoms or sweat pants are ideal because they reduce the friction of your thighs. The actual motion of power walking is a swing of the hips to account for the longer gate. It's because of this that joggers put far more pressure on their knees than walkers do – they bounce on their joints as they jog which is bad for the bones, whereas walkers walk with a horizontal movement, gliding forward across the ground. A good way to walk faster and therefore burn more fat is to pump your arms with each stride, as your hormones will burn far more fat when you engage your abs and buttocks at the same time.

Once You Start, It's Easy to Keep Going

Because your mood and general sense of well-being will be dramatically increased by partaking in this low-impact exercise, you'll find that instead of it feeling like a chore to carry on, you will instead find that quitting is the last thing on your mind. The new effective weight loss that comes with taking on this exercise will mean that your goal will be a lot clearer and instead of feeling like you are forcing yourself to do it, you will feel as though you are being pleasantly pulled towards it. When people take on walking for weight loss they discover that reaching their target of 10,000 steps is both exciting and satisfying. The goals are measurable, and therefore relatively easy to carry through. The increased morale and feeling of accomplishment will mean that other fitness goals will seem a lot easier to tackle. It just takes a couple of weeks to create a habit that gives you the results you've always wanted, and the results in turn will make it easy to keep up it.

Why Pre-Walk Stretching & Walking Gear Is Important

You can quite literally not only change your body shape but also change your life by walking 10,000 steps each time you walk for exercise. However, walking to burn fat is actually quite different to walking for the purpose of getting from one place to another. Your legs, abs and buttocks all have the potential to shed pounds and get in shape – and so to get the results you desire, preparing your body with stretching and getting properly dressed beforehand will bring you greater results.

Footwear

Walking is a low-impact activity on your body, but because you will be walking 10,000 steps it's a good idea to wear the correct footwear to ensure your feet are comfortable and protected. The two activities of walking and running are quite different; therefore walking shoes can alter greatly from running shoes. The reason for this is because our joints and muscles move in different ways during these activities, so a different type of support is needed. When people run they bend their knees at a larger angle than when they walk, as opposed to the horizontal fluid motion of walking. The best type of shoe for advanced walking or power walking is one with a lot of cushioning, as well as being light in weight. Feet can swell when walking 10,000 steps, so they should be roomy and flexible enough to accommodate this. When walking, we naturally touch the ground first with our heel and then roll through to push off with our toes – so it's good to get a shoe that is flexible in the middle to absorb each step.

Let the Steps Be Counted For You

Probably the best investment you'll make when taking up walking for weight loss is a pedometer, for it will do all the step counting for you. Because leg length determines the distance it will take to perform 10,000 steps, a pedometer will take all the guess work out. It will also help to push you further because it will help you determine your maximum distance and speed. The three main types of pedometer that are used are accelerometers, coiled spring devices and hairspring models. Hairspring ones need to be kept in a constant upright position so are not very reliable when it comes to walking 10,000 steps. If you go for a more high-end pedometer you'll be able to enjoy the benefits of very accurate readings, as these can be work on the wrist and will count the number of steps no matter which direction they are held. Other benefits of these devices are speed estimates, heart rate monitoring and calorie burning information. You don't have to spend a lot or get the latest model, but you should make sure it's a durable one that will help you get a decent amount of data so that you can continue to move forward and reach your goals.

How to Avoid Chaffing

Friction can be a big issue for walkers. It depends on your body shape, but shorts could cause you to chaff your inner thigh area. A good prevention for this is investing in some good workout pants – make sure the material allows for minimal thigh friction as well as being loose enough to allow a good flow of air. It's possible to buy some that actually wick sweat away so that you'll always stay dry during a walk.

Stretching

Even though the act of walking is relatively stress-free on you body, it is still possible to sustain an injury doing so, so stretching before you head out is a very good idea. Starting at the top of your body, work your way down until each major muscle group has been limbered up. This is the best order: neck, then shoulders, then mid back, then lower back, then hips, then buttocks, then thighs, then calves. Finally, stretch your ankles carefully by rolling them in small circles.

A couple of things to look out for and avoid when stretching are not to over extend the knees. Stretching them beyond a ninety degree angle is too far and will do more harm than good. Also, pulsing whilst stretching is not a good idea because a constant flow of oxygen is needed in order to loosen up your muscles. So, lean into the stretch as far as you can whilst breathing deeply and steadily. The act of pushing into the stretch after a long exhale will improve the elasticity of your muscles.

With the right mind-set, you can stay positive and proactive in your eating and exercise habits to both dramatically increase and improve your health and fitness levels.

~~~

POWER WALKING – HOW TO BURN BELLY FAT BY WALKING 10,000 STEPS (& EATING POWERFUL NUTRIENTS)

Introduction

When it comes to power walking it's reassuring to know that your long-term success will be gained in a short period of time just by perseverance. You will be able to drop those unwanted pounds from the midsection, gain a great metabolism that won't let you down and build lean muscle, all from power walking. This book will also give you food tips on the best nutrients that will optimise your hard work, and make sure you get the most out of it. Not only this, but anxiety and stress will be relieved due to your body's natural endorphins that are released as your serotonin levels are boosted by your efforts. All you need to do, is take those first steps and you'll find that it is not willpower driving you but rather 'want power' pulling you towards your goal.

Let's Achieve Those Goals

In order to achieve our goals, we first need to know what they are. This is vital in order for us to succeed, so we can be realistic about the weight we want to be and set our expectations accordingly. So instead of being unrealistic, let's set achievable goals that will not only allow you to drop pounds from your waist, but also improve your overall health and eating habits. Your goals don't have to be amazingly complex, as long as you're specific about how you visualise your long-term result. For example, they could be increasing your muscle mass, dropping pounds and then maintaining the body shape you desire, or lowering your blood pressure. Instead of being short sporadic efforts that do not have longevity, these efforts require gradual and sustainable changes to your life habits.

Significant Milestones

If you set yourself small milestones to achieve, as you achieve them they will bring you a step closer to your desired result, and allow you to reach your goal. So, dropping 10 pounds can be a small milestone that will bring you closer to your end goal of maintaining a lower body weight - just make sure you give yourself time to achieve this. As you go along, your strength and endurance will increase and then you will be able to re-evaluate your small milestones to make your workouts more intense and even more rewarding. For example, walking further distances and walking with small hand weights will burn the fat a lot more quickly.

What You Need For Success

A vital part in helping you achieve weight loss by walking, is having the correct equipment for your workouts. Comfortable walking shoes that provide good arch support, a multi-functioning pedometer and a journal to record your achievements are all important. Realistically, you will need to build up to walking 10,000 steps per day. So a good thing to do is create realistic small milestones that will bring you closer to that 10,000 steps per day. Mark down in your journal the small achievements as you achieve them because this will give you a great feeling of accomplishment.

How To Use Positive Reinforcement

When you see changes in yourself, your body and your weight, mark them down in your journal especially when they are unexpected. Some great changes that you may notice could be increased muscle tone, feeling less stressed, getting a better night's sleep, or feeling younger. Whatever they are, marking them down and acknowledging them will benefit you greatly and increase your commitment levels.

The Positive Effects of Walking

There are many benefits of walking for weight loss that many of us at first don't realise. When you see these changes and take note of them you are much more likely to stick with it, because you see how walking can really alter your body shape and boost your health. Power walking is a great form of cardiovascular exercise and strength training combined, and is low-impact on the body and joints. Other health benefits are keeping age-related diseases away, reduced belly fat, reducing your stress or anxiety, deterring heart disease and dropping pounds. Although walking for weight loss is designed to drop pounds, try to remember that your efforts are also changing your life and restructuring your life habits. By remembering this you can absolutely stay proactive and positive in striving to reach your milestones, and this is a great mind-set to have.

How To Optimise Fat Burning By Power Walking

Although it may be tempting to progress from walking to jogging or running, these exercises can actually be more detrimental because they can directly affect your knees and joints due to the way you bounce off the floor as you jog or run. Power walking is a much better alternative and here's why: it has great benefits such as taking less time to burn off fat and calories, improved thought processes and improved brain functioning, but it is also a low-stress exercise that is easy on your joints due to the gliding movement of the power walker. In next to no time you'll be looking better and there's no need to worry about getting injured whilst doing it.

Selecting The Right Footwear

Because power walking requires pushing your body harder than normal walking, it's important to have the right shoes. It's a little-known fact that power walkers actually walk the same speed as joggers, however joggers hit the floor with twice as much force. The body mechanics between the two are very different, as real progress in power walking is achieved by the walker pumping their arms, both engaging the abdomen and clenching the buttocks therefore gliding horizontally in a graceful motion. When done correctly, the abdomen remaining tense throughout the walk and this will ensure that it becomes toned and sheds pounds from the midsection.

So, select footwear that is both flexible and allows for good motion in the middle range of the foot by giving good arch support. To avoid strain in the heels and the shins stay away from flat and hard souls that don't have much flexibility. Because power walking requires long even strides, flexibility is key in selecting footwear for advanced walking.

When it comes to footwear it is also important to make sure that they are made with natural wicking materials. This will give you the ventilation when you sweat, and you should be aware that shoes you need for power walking is quite different to the shoes that you need for jogging or running.

To avoid chaffing and unwanted friction when power walking it is very important that you select the appropriate pants that are both comfortable and flexible. Most tracksuit bottoms or work-out pants will be fine for power walking, and as you build-up speed you make sure that they remain comfortable.

Before You Set Out

Take a little bit of time to gradually build up to a good pace rather than just setting out at your fastest speed as it usually takes about 5 to 10 minutes to get your muscles fully warmed up. So, after a couple of minutes stop and stretch your shoulders, arms and hamstrings, then while keeping your hips still stretch your waist by bending the upper torso to each side. Unlike normal walking, power walking is absolutely a full body exercise therefore you should stretch from your head all the way down to your toes before you embark on the main portion of your walk.

Total Body Conditioning

The major muscle groups become toned and firmed up during this type of walking because it requires people to use all of their muscles. To burn the maximum amount of fat and calories when power walking, always engage your core muscles. You can do this by imagining there is a string attached to your midsection and someone who is taller than you is standing behind you and pulling the string thereby drawing your stomach up and back. So when you draw your navel up and in, your core muscles will be totally engaged throughout your walk. Keep this up for the duration of your power walk, and you'll see major changes in the conditioning and toning of your stomach.

Like everything, this will become easier as time goes on, as when you first try it it may be hard to keep your abs engaged the whole time. The muscles at the sides of your torso (your obliques), will be engaged by your opposite arm and leg movements while you walk, so the combined motion of your limbs as you stride will give your torso good muscle tone.

As well as focusing on your abs, make sure your buttocks are engaged for the duration of the walk. The combination of tightening up your abs and buttocks is what turns this cardio exercise into a genuine strength training exercise, which results in maximising the amount of calories you burn. Lean muscle will be developed even when walking horizontally across a flat plain as your body burns calories, and therefore you will see a dramatic increase in your metabolism.

Why You Should Walk 4.5 Miles Per Hour

Not dissimilar to the speed of jogging, the target speed of 4.5 mph is perfect for power walking. Try to make sure your strides are long and even and focus on matching your leg movements with your arm movements, as when performed properly there should be a slight but easy sway to your hips. This will allow you to reach greater speeds with ease, but make sure this doesn't break into a slow run. This is because when you jog or run you are performing both vertical and horizontal movements, and when you're power walking you should only be striding horizontally, not bouncing off the ground at all. If you find yourself doing this, just slow down a little bit and adjust your stride accordingly because maintaining good form is very beneficial when it comes to shedding pounds from walking.

When walking at a moderate and slow pace it is rare to feel out of breath or break a sweat, due to it being a moderate impact activity. And although it can burn a lot of calories and get rid of fat it doesn't have much effect on your respiratory system or cardio. But when you up the ante to power walking, the first few times it's normal to feel knackered and winded. So during the first few times you power walk listen to your body and pay attention to how it feels now that you have boosted your walking speed. Think about how your shoes feel and think about which areas of your body are struggling, and if your hips start to ache you could always take the activity to a shock absorbing surface like a track. Your ankles and knees should feel fine if you're power walking correctly, but your hips may start to hurt when you first attempt it and that is when you can possibly try a different surface.

How To Reach Faster Speeds Consistently

This is the easiest way to work out your speed: know how far you're walking and how long it takes to get there, then divide the walking distance by the number of hours that it takes you to walk this far and this will equal the number of miles per hour you are travelling. So, from the outset try to walk for one full hour, and due to the moderate impact of the exercise you're not likely to experience any injury or bodily stress.

To get your speed up, the best way is to pump your arms harder and faster, because then your legs will follow. The reason why you use your arms to gain speed is because if you focus on your legs then your buttocks may begin to experience a burning sensation. You may not need to train for a full hour given that you can burn more calories in less time with power walking. But if you can manage it, you get a lot more benefits such as a greater release of endorphins and a greater amount of stress relief as well as emotional, physical and mental benefits. It's easier to walk for longer than jog or run because of the relative ease of this activity even if the exercise is pretty new to you. You could always stop for a moment to get your breath back and then go harder once to energy has regained.

To get to the 4.5 per hour pace, you need to build up to it as this means you will be power walking a whole mile in about 30 min which isn't going to be easy straightaway. So, instead of trying to go to full-on and then burning out after a few minutes, pushing your body to go longer while simultaneously using the correct form will give you way better results. Because at a speed of about 4.5 mph you can burn off just over 200 calories in only half an hour, and this can be better than jogging because you're using the same amount of energy either way. You'll notice great improvements in your target speed by holding a small pair of handheld weights or by strapping on some ankle weights, as this will push you way beyond just improving the speed of your walking. There are also benefits of doing this exercise indoors if the weather is bad, such as using a treadmill because it will give you the option of altering the incline of the walking service to increase the challenge therefore burning more calories.

Why You Shouldn't Always Walk At Your Fastest Pace

When walking for an entire hour, the best way to minimise your risk of physical injury is a power walking plan where you can gradually increase in speed, with a period of peak speed and then gradually slow down at the end. You shouldn't come to a sudden standstill at the end of the hour, and you shouldn't start out with big quick strides. So, at the end of the exercise spend at least 10 minutes bringing your body back down to a steady pace slowly. Your breathing should return to normal and your heart should be beating slowly by the time you have stopped walking. When you're ready for your post-workout stretching, your muscles will be feeling warm and ready for it. You should focus on doing the same stretch routine you did during the warm-up, but make sure you add in your abs and buttocks as this will give you the whole body post-workout stretch routine that you need.

The Psychological Benefits of Power Walking

When walking at optimal speeds, not only will your body reward you for your efforts but your brain will too. Benefits include de-cluttering your mind, de-stressing, and giving you a stimulating rush of endorphins. Indeed, you will also have increased levels of inner calm and peace as this activity allows for introspection Studies have shown that regular walking improves sleep and helps to slow mental decline considerably. It also helps by focussing on breathing and other basic and automatic functions whilst clearing the brain of external stressors as it is the ideal opportunity to operate with meditative intent. So, if dropping pounds isn't enough motivation for you, think about your overall well-being, less anxiety or depression and having a far greater energy as benefits worth aiming for.

Nutrition and Power Walking - What You Should Eat and Why

It is absolutely possible to shed pounds in just the first couple of weeks of power walking, as it is a great combination of both strength training and cardio exercise, so you'll be able to visually see the difference in your body. But if you want to really make the most of your hard work and optimise your results, you can add a good diet plan. So work to fuel your body with a great array of powerful nutrients instead of completely focusing on cutting calories alone. Here's how.

The Best Foods

You'll be building new lean muscle from power walking and if you need a bit of extra fuel your metabolism can burn off more fat and calories. This can easily be done with strength training. Foods with a lot of protein will always be the best thing to consume if you want to increase lean muscle because protein is the only thing the builds lean muscle. Carbs and fats are energy sources whereas protein is vital in increasing your metabolism and maintaining lean muscle. So feed your body what it needs to regenerate and rebuild the targeted muscle groups after a power walking routine by eating the right high protein foods. Natural food sources are always the best way to go when getting essential nutrients, and this is preferable above supplements that some people rely on. This is because the body finds it easier to break down and recognise protein in this form - even some of the highest quality supplements won't be fully be absorbed by the body and what the body can't use it just get rid of.

As well as the obvious choices of white meat, fish and other animal derived protein, there is also the great option of true nuts such as walnuts, pecans and almonds as these are optimal sources of protein. Almond butter and nut butters are also optimal sources of protein, but steer clear of peanuts as they are not a true nut and are packed with way more starch so will be detrimental to your walking for weight loss goal.

Other good sources of protein are chickpeas, lentils, pinto beans, kidney beans, red beans, and black beans as these are low in fat and high in protein. They can easily be made into a tasty soup and other dishes to power up after a workout and replenish your body. They are also easy on the wallet and due to them being very high in protein they are also rich in magnesium, fibre, iron and potassium. They increase and improve your digestive regularity, improve your heart health and they can increase your collagen production. So by adding these to your diet you can avoid many health risks whilst simultaneously building muscle. By improving your diet with their protein dense nature you will also reduce the risk of physical injury. They are also very filling so there's not much chance of going hungry and lacking energy.

The best meats when it comes to protein is white meats such as fish, chicken and turkey breast because they are full of nutrients and can be a good base for soups, pasta and salad. Several servings per week will help you gain lean muscle but be careful of your fish supplier due to increased mercury levels.

Which Foods Will Give You The Most Energy

The most essential foods for maintaining a high level of energy when power walking are carbohydrates. When selecting the right carbohydrates, be aware of the huge difference between natural sources of carbohydrates that give the body energy and nourishment versus those that are heavily refined. These have a bad reputation due to the major weight gain that is possible by consuming too much of them.

Other sources of fuel that are good can come in the form of vegetables and fresh fruits as these are water dense, are rich in nourishment, rich in vitamins and overall are low in calories. When maintaining your walking for weight loss exercise plan, minimising the amount of empty calorie foods you consume is vital. This is because these foods have been stripped of almost all of their nutritional benefits. White flour is one example to stay away from, because when consumed these carbs are converted into sugars in no time, and therefore can be detrimental to your internal organ systems as well as increasing your risk of other nutrition related health problems. When it comes to grains, products that are offered in the closest form of their natural state are the ones that you should always go for.

A good way to help regulate your blood sugar levels and get rid of bad toxins from your blood flow is to eat steel cut oatmeal. This decreases your risk of developing diabetes and adding cinnamon makes it tasty. Consuming hot oatmeal with chopped fruit such as blackberries, blueberries or any other unprocessed nutritional fruit will give a good boost to your health. You can also add nuts into this mix, pecans being a good choice as they are able to provide the body with an added rich dose of protein. This kind of meal is really beneficial to the heart and one that will absolutely give you the energy that is needed to maintain a gruelling one hour power walking session.

A Well-Balanced Blend of Essential Food Groups Is Key

A lot of the reasons why people develop weight loss issues is by not sticking to good habits when it comes to eating. Some diet plans are also missing a lot of ingredients that require balance. There is good and bad fat - when people pursue too much of bad fat along with too many refined carbs it becomes a downward spiral to weight gain. And when they try to compensate by swinging in the opposite way, they often cut out major food groups like carbohydrates entirely. Carbohydrates are needed in order to represent a well-balanced blend of all the essential food groups. So instead of dropping pounds fast they are actually denying their bodies important powerful nutrients that will benefit them in their exercise regime.

Although cutting out carbohydrates entirely can absolutely help you drop pounds, these types of diets don't last long and the reason why is because as soon as the individual returns to their old eating habits, the lost weight will return rapidly. Cutting out carbohydrates entirely causes the metabolism to slow down, so it's always a good idea to give your body the nutrients it needs. Sticking to roughly 2000 calories per day will help you reach a healthy weight more quickly than anything else, and once there it will be far easier to maintain it.

Fresh Is Best

When snacking, the best way to reduce unwanted calories is to always eat fresh. You get a rush of natural energy by eating an apple as well as keeping your teeth clean, likewise a handful of sugar snow peas will give you three times the recommended daily amount of vitamin C that your body needs. So, absolutely stay clear of chips, cookies, cakes, and processed sandwich bread as these foods will contain an unhealthy amount of calories, sodium, sugar and fat and will provide no benefit to your body, so don't rely on them. Another benefit of vegetables and fresh fruits are that they are very dense in fibre as well as being filled with water, and this is important after a power walking regime as they will replenish your stores thereby minimising the amount of water that you need to drink in order to stay hydrated.

Good Oil and Bad Fats

It's a good idea to limit the amount of cream, cheese and butter you consume as part of your regular diet as these dairy products contain a lot of fat. Instead, get healthy fats from fish, olives and nuts. The best cooking oil is coconut due to its antibacterial properties as well as being able to be heated at high heats without chemically changing due to its stable nature. Try to avoid olive oil - even though it has the reputation of being the best oil for a healthy diet, it's actually highly unstable and the composition of its chemicals change once it is heated, so it's therefore greatly inferior to coconut oil. Cold it's fine though on salads, but avoid it when it comes to boiling of frying.

It's recommended that you should try to eat at least one full tablespoon of coconut oil per day as this will be of great benefit to your diet. It has vital nutrients that help brain functioning, as well as lowering acidity levels in people who have routinely consumed a lot of alcohol or who have previously had a high sugar diet. This helps accelerate weight loss on the stomach and you can use this oil instead of butter by using it in your dishes and it can also be used in beverages and soups.

The Benefits of Fresh Pure Water

An important part of weight loss is choosing the right kind of drinks, as this is just as important as giving your body the right types of fats. Sports drinks, even low-calorie ones, can be tempting to consume as they boast to give you optimal hydration. However these actually do more harm than good when it comes to your efforts to drop pounds. This is because they are packed with a lot of sweeteners and sodium, so with a lot of food colouring and unhealthy sugars added they actually detrimental to what you're trying to achieve. Taking this into account, there is no better alternative than pure fresh water. And although some people like to say that water is too plain on the taste buds, you can easily add a slice of lemon or lime to dramatically change the flavour. Another way to increase your metabolism and regulate your blood pressure can be to add a few sprinkles of cayenne pepper to a tall grass and warm or cold water.

Amazingly, drinking green tea instead of coffee, as long as it is unsweetened, can actually give you as much as five pounds of weight loss in one week. So when you find it hard to shed those last few pounds take this into consideration for its possibly drastic positive outcome. When it comes to caffeine in general, it is a good idea to heavily limit your intake. This includes all sodas, including diet soda as this has been proven to be just as bad for your body is the full sugar types, so to make the most of your workout and get the best results, go for pure fruit juice. Similarly to low-fat milk, you can consume several ounces of these per day and they will help add useful nutrients to your diet. It's fine to have one coffee in the morning - just go easy on the amount of sugar and cream that you have with it.

Why Snacking Can Help You In The Long-Run

It may be hard to believe, but dark chocolate is actually good for you. In fact, it is recommended as part of your regular walking for weight loss program as it can dramatically boost your serotonin levels. It's a guilt-free way to indulge in a tasty snack, whilst reducing your food cravings, therefore helping to diet in the long-run. So it's true that some of the most beneficial foods are some of the most tasty. So, denying your sweet tooth of chocolate entirely is actually worse for you overall as it has been proven that people who eat dark chocolate tend to eat a lot less than those that deny themselves of it entirely. It just goes to show that adding powerful nutrients can have its good moments. So when you feel lacking in motivation when it comes to your power walking for weight loss plan, an easy and quick way to get back your drive and lift your spirits is to indulge in a couple of rich squares of dark - keeping your hunger at bay in the process.

~~~